THE GUIDE TO NUTRITION AND DIET FOR DIALYSIS PATIENTS

Dr. Shuang Chen

ISBN: 978-1-60594-026-7

Printed in the United States of America by Llumina Press

Library of Congress Control Number: 2008924096

DEDICATION

Dedicated to Dr. Peng Fu, Dr. Jing Xu, Dr. Caobo Feng, Nurse Ms. Hong Su, Nurse Ms. Yuan Wan, and Nurse Ms. Lili Liao in Changhai Hospital, Shanghai who are treating my father with professionalism.

To my ill father, without whom none of this would have happened.

To my dear mother, who takes care of my father wholeheartedly every single day.

To my brothers Qisu and Weiwei, who aid our parents wonderfully.

THE GUIDE TO NUTRITION AND DIET FOR DIALYSIS PATIENTS

Shuang Chen, M.D., R.H.(AHG)
Donglian Cai, M.D.

1. What is hemodialysis? (abbreviation "HD")

Hemodialysis, often called simply, dialysis, is a therapy to cleanse the blood of impurities when the kidneys can no longer perform this vital function. Hemodialysis uses a semipermeable membrane to eliminate wastes and excessive electrolytes from the blood, and thus prevent the fatal danger caused by uremia, the collection of excessive urea, creatinine, and other nitrogen-containing substances in the blood.

There are three types of hemodialyzers: composite fiber module, multilayer module, and coil module. By moving across a dialysis membrane, the amount of water, electrolytes, urea, creatinine, and glucose in the blood can be controlled. This kind of dialysis will not decrease the amount of blood cells nor the protein in the blood. Hemodialysis can reverse body fluid retention and help prevent hypertension (high blood pressure) and hyperkalemia (excessive potassium in the blood). It is also helpful for maintaining normal serum electrolyte levels. However, hemodialysis can also cause the loss of some vitamins and hormones from the human body. Nevertheless, hemodialysis is generally beneficial to patients for improving the symptoms of renal (kidney) failure, prolonging life, and promoting the quality of life.

2. What is peritoneal dialysis (abbreviation "PD")?

The word "peritoneal" refers to the membrane lining the abdomen and pelvic area. It encloses such major organs as the liver, stomach, colon, and small intestine. Peritoneal dialysis is the process of transforming and exchanging water and solute between the peritoneal dialysate (the material being passed through the membrane) in the peritoneal cavity and the blood in peritoneal capillaries by moving the dialysate through the peritoneum, a natural biological membrane. Peritoneal dialysate includes sodium, chloride, lactate, and high concentration glucose leading to osmotic pressure. On the other hand, end stage renal disease patients carry a number of toxic substances in their blood, such as creatinine and urea. Peritoneal dialysis uses the properties of the peritoneum, a semipermeable membrane, to exchange substances, in order to eliminate water and metabolic wastes and to supply alkaline base. Peritoneal dialysis uses three principles: diffusion, ultrafiltration, and absorption. The two most common types of peritoneal dialysis are continuous ambulatory peritoneal dialysis (CAPD) and automatic peritoneal dialysis.

3. **What are the principles of a healthy diet for the hemodialysis patient?**

(1) Equilibrium of dietary nutrition:
The nutrients include carbohydrates, saccharide, fat, protein, vitamins, minerals, and trace elements. It is very important to eat the above nutrients in a balanced diet every day. An example of daily diet for an adult of 120-130 pounds (55-60 kg) is shown on the next page.

Type	Food	Weight (Grams)	Serving	Calories (Kilocalories)	Protein (Grams)	Water (Milliliters)
Carbohydrate	Rice	400	One full bowl per time	628	11.6	251
	Potato	40	Half potato, one-third of sweet potato	31	0.8	32
	Sugar Jam	50 15	Six British teaspoons One British teaspoon	224	0.1	6
Protein	Fish	80	One small fish or one piece of thick fish fillet	116	14.9	58
	Meat	80	Lean beef, pork or chicken	101	18.0	60
	Egg	50	One egg	81	6.2	37
	Tofu	100	Three table-spoons of yellow bean, one-third cube of tofu	77	6.8	87
	Milk	100	Half cup	59	2.9	89
Fat	Cooking Oil	60	Five ~ six British teaspoons	530	0	0
Minerals/ Vitamins	Vegetable	200	Varies by vegetable	52	3.2	184
	Fruit	50	One apple or one pear. (Choose low potassium fruit)	41	0.3	39
	Mushroom Seaweed	Proper amount				
Other	Noodle	60	Noodle, won-ton, bread,. or bun	222	5.4	60
Total				2162	70.2	849

Note 1 : One tablespoon = 15 milliliters

One full bowl = 480 grams

One British teaspoon=10 milliliters

One cup =200 milliliters

Note 2: This table is not suitable for diabetes patients and end-stage renal disease patients.

Note 3: Foods listed in the table above are only a suggestion for patients.

(2) Proper high-quality protein

The proper amount of high-quality protein is based on a patient's age, body shape, and weight. The proper amount of high-quality protein for hemodialysis patients is 1.0-2.0 gram/kilogram of body weight per day. The supplemental amount of protein should not be less or more than this recommendation. Too much protein may increase the level of urea, nitrogen, and potassium in the blood. Too little protein may result in malnutrition or anemia. Eggs, milk, meat, fish, shellfish, and soy products are the best sources of high-quality protein. The intake of this protein should be balanced in the meals.

(3) Supplement of calories

When the human body does not have sufficient energy, it will obtain the supplementary amount needed by consuming bodily protein. This will cause a drop in energy as the result of increasing levels of waste (such as decomposition substances, creatinine in the blood, and urea nitrogen). In addition, even with sufficient protein intake, it will be used to generate energy when lacking of sufficient calories. Therefore, it is very important to consume the proper amount of saccharide and fat in order to provide sufficient energy. Nevertheless, diabetic patients should strictly limit the intake of sugar and food containing sugar. The intake of calories by hemodialysis patients should be controlled at 35-40 kilocalories/kilogram of body weight per day.

(4) Limiting intake of salt

The intake of salt by hemodialysis patients should be limited to less than 2 grams daily. Do not eat food processed with salt, such as salted vegetables, pickles, salted seafood, pickled fish, canned fish, salted meat, sausage, ham, smoked sausage, smoked fish, preserved meat, butter, butter substitutes, cheese, bread, (French bread and other breads), and various seasonings, including any brand of soy sauce.

Please refer to *Appendix Four* to find out what kinds of food are high in sodium. Please refer to the additional text below for a discussion of the disadvantages of excessive salt intake.

(5) Restricting intake of potassium

Due to renal failure and decreased urine output, dialysis patients cannot maintain the normal level of potassium in the blood. There will be an increase of blood potassium level (hyperkalemia) leading to an adverse influence on cardiac and cerebrovascular functions. To prevent hyperkalemia, patients who undergo dialysis three times a week should limit their intake of potassium to 1300 mg daily.

(6) Strict control of excessive water intake

For a discussion of the threat of excessive water intake, please refer to the following text.

Among the above six principles, the restrictions on water and salt intake are especially important and cannot be neglected. These principles can greatly affect a dialysis patient's longevity, as well as their quality of living.

4. What are the principles of diet for peritoneal dialysis patients?

The principles of balanced nutrition, proper energy supplement, and limiting salt intake are basically the same as those for hemodialysis patients. However, peritoneal dialysis patients can eat an additional quantity of high quality protein (also known as high biological valence, or value, protein), for example, 1.2~1.5 grams/kilogram of body weight per day. Peritoneal dialysis patients are not restrained in their potassium intake. They can also have greater fluid intake compared with the strict limitation for hemodialysis patients.

5. Why do hemodialysis patients have to check their weight every day?

Patients with chronic renal failure undergoing continuous dialysis usually have symptoms of diminished urine output (oliguria) or complete suppression of urine secretion by the kidneys (anuria). Therefore, water intake should be strictly controlled because edema, hypertension, and even heart failure may occur. Hemodialysis patients have to check their weight every day in order to know the balance of their body fluids. During dialysis treatment, the increase in the patient's weight should not exceed 1 to 1.5 kilograms. This also provides a basis for patients and their family when calculating daily water intake.

6. Why is it necessary to limit the intake of water and salt ?

During hemodialysis treatment, the most important factor in the patient's diet is to strictly control daily water and salt intake. This will protect cardiac and vascular function and promote a better quality of life and even prolong life. Patients will feel thirsty if they eat too much salt, and drinking too much water will result in weight gain, and furthermore, lead to edema, increased blood pressure, and even pulmonary edema. Under severe conditions, it may also cause heart failure. When pulmonary edema and heart failure occur, patients will experience trouble breathing (dyspnea), asthma, and anxiety, and will have additional difficulty in breathing when lying down.

7. How should the hemodialysis patient control daily water intake?

Patients who undergo hemodialysis once a week normally need to supplement their water intake by 100 ml water plus the amount of total urine output in the previous 24 hours. For example, for a patient whose total urine output from the previous day was 1000 ml, the water supplement for the next day should be limited to 1000 + 100 = 1100 ml.

The daily water supplement for patients undergoing hemodialysis twice a week is 300 ml plus the amount of total urine output in the previous 24 hours. For instance, if total urine output yesterday was 1000 ml, today's water supplement should be limited to 1000 + 300 = 1300 ml.

For patients who undergo hemodialysis three times a week, the daily water supplement should be 500 ml plus the amount of total urine output during last 24 hours. For example, if total urine output for the previous days was 1000 ml for the previous day, the next day's water supplement should be limited to 1000 + 500 = 1500 ml.

If a patient had no urine output over the past 24 hours, the water supplement should not exceed 500 ml.(Patients and their families will received training at the dialysis canter in how to measure daily urine output.)

8. Some patients believe that it is fine to drink more water because dialysis can "eliminate" excessive liquid. Is this correct?

No. Hemodialysis patients cannot rely on the ultrafiltration of dialysis to eliminate excessive body water. This is so because rapid and large quantity of water eliminated by ultrafiltration during hemodialysis will cause symptoms such as drop in blood pressure, muscle cramps, and headache. In addition, long-term water overloading will increase cardiovascular loading and lead to serious consequences.

9. In addition to drinking water, coffee, and tea, what other liquids also contain water?

Among these are wine and alcoholic drinks, soup, various sauces, juices, ice cream, jams and jellies, milk, soy milk, porridge, rice, liquid medications, liquid vitamins, and carbonated beverages, as well as the water taken with medicine and ice consumed as part of the diet.

10. What kinds of drinking habit should patients develop?

Hemodialysis patients should develop good drinking habits, as follows: **(1)** Do not drink when you are not thirsty, and avoid having a second sip when you can be satisfied with only one; **(2)** drink from a small glass or cup; **(3)** before eating canned food, dispose of whatever liquid is in the can; **(4)** keep yourself busy to help you forget the desire to drink; **(5)** if you like to drink extra cold water, put the water in a refrigerator to cool it down instead of using ice; **(6)** replace water with soup to swallow medicine taken after meals; **(7)** do not drink unfamiliar mineral water.

What kinds of food are high in sodium？

(1) Processed foods, such as pickled foods, smoked sausage, sausage, ham, pickled meat, salty vegetables, pickled vegetable, and kimchi.**(2)** Canned foods. **(3)** Fast food. **(4)** Snacks, such as popcorn and potato chips (Make sure to check the ingredient tables on the package so that the amount of sodium does not exceed 300 mg). **(5)** All kinds of bottled seasonings and sauces. **(6)** Frozen foods.

For a detailed list, please refer to *Appendix Four*, "High Sodium Foods"

    a. Choose salt substitute as often as possible when cooking (Need to check sodium level.)

b. When dining out, request that the restaurant not season your food with salt, and ask for light soy sauce (can be diluted with water) or other low-salted seasoning so that you can control your sodium intake.

c. Read nutrition facts on the packaging label before making any purchase at the market.

d. Do not purchase food that lists sodium as the first ingredient on its label.

12. What kinds of spice and herb should dialysis patients use instead of salt to add flavor?

All spices. Use with beef, fish, beets, cabbage, carrots, peas, and fruit.

Basil. Use with beef, pork, and most vegetables.

Bay Leaf. Use with beef, pork, and most vegetables.

Caraway. Use with beef, pork, green beans, cauliflower, cabbage, beets, and asparagus.

Cardamom. Use with fruit and in baked foods.

Curry. Use with beef, chicken, pork, fish, green beans, and carrots and in marinades.

Dill. Use with beef, chicken, green beans, cabbage, carrots, and peas, and in dips.

Ginger, Use with beef, chicken, pork, green beans, cauliflower, and eggplant.

Marjoram. Use with beef, chicken, pork, green beans, cauliflower and eggplant.

Rosemary. Use with chicken, pork, cauliflower, and peas, and in marinades.

Thyme. Use with beef, pork, chicken, fish, green beans, beets and carrots.

Sage. Use with chicken, pork, and eggplant, and in salad dressings.

Tarragon. Use with fish, asparagus, beets, cabbage, and cauliflower and in marinades.

13. How should these spices and herbs be used?

Below are tips for cooking with herbs and spices as a salt-substitute flavoring:

    a. Purchase spices and herbs in small amounts. When they sit on the shelf for years, they lose their flavor.

    b. Use no more than ¼ teaspoon of dried spices (3/4 of a teaspoon of fresh spices) per pound of meat.

    c. Add ground spices to the food about 15 minutes before the end of the cooking period.

    d. Add whole spices to food at least one hour before the end of the cooking period.

    e. Combine herbs with oil or butter, let set for 30 minutes to bring out the flavor of the herb, and then brush on foods while they cook, or brush meat with oil and sprinkle on herbs one hour before cooking.

f. Crush dried herbs before adding to foods.

14. Do most salt substitutes contain potassium?

Yes. If a dialysis patient is on a potassium-restricted diet, he or she must be very cautious in using salt substitutes because most of them contain some form of potassium. Check with your doctor or dietitian before using any salt substitute. However, in patients with a low potassium level, the salt substitute containing potassium may exactly match his or her needs.

15. What if the patient has a high cholesterol level?

Changing this patient's diet may help lower the cholesterol level in his or her blood. A dietitian will recommend the kinds of fat and animal foods to be eaten. Also, the patient's doctor may prescribe a special medication to reduce the blood cholesterol level.

16. What if the patient has diabetes?

A patient suffering from diabetic end-stage renal disease undergoing dialysis should keeps observe strict limitations on his/her diet plan.

A dietitian will help to develop a meal plan particularly for such patients.

17. Is there any thing else the patient should know about diet while undergoing dialysis?

The following tips can be highly helpful with your diet:

a. Fresh or plain frozen vegetables contain no added salt. Drain all the cooking fluid from canned vegetables before serving.

b. Canned fruits usually contain less potassium than fresh fruits.
Drain all the fluid before serving.

c. Non-dairy creamers are low in phosphorus and can be used in place of milk.

d. The label on food packages will provide information about any of the ingredients that may not be allowed in the patient's diet. Learn to read these labels carefully.

e. To avoid salt, many herbs and spices can be used to make the patient's diet more interesting. Check with a dietitian for a list of useful herbs and spices.

18. How do I control or diminish feelings of thirst?

a. For patients with diabetes, make sure to control the blood sugar level. The higher the blood sugar level, the more likely is the thirst for liquids.

b. Avoid eating sweets.

c. Brush your teeth or gargle to relieve mild thirst.

d. Avoid expose under the sun for long periods

e. Holding a slice of lemon in the mouth can quench thirst.

f. Stay on a low sodium diet. Restrict daily salt intake to less than 2g.

g. Holding a small piece of ice in the mouth relieves thirst because ice can retain water longer than liquid water.

h. Non-diabetic patients can quench their thirst by eating sour plums or by chewing gum. Patients with diabetes can chew sugar-free gum to relieve thirst.

i. Refrigerating fruit before eating it will relieve thirst more than eating fruit kept under normal temperature. Patients with diabetes should eat fruit low in sugar, such as grapefruit, papaya, carambola, lemons, platinum melon, mango melon, honeydew melon, Huanghemi melon, lingmi melon, Jingta temple melon, apples, small oranges, plums, apricots, plum cot, golden red peaches, other peaches, pears, and tough pears.

j. Applying jam or margarine when eating multiple-grained bread or wheat bread can relieve thirst (patients with diabetes should not eat jam.)

19. How does one judge if a hemodialysis patient's body fluid level has reached relative balance?

The method is based on monitoring the patient's DRY WEIGHT every day. For example, if a patient weighs 80 kilograms before dialysis whereas his normal weight is 78.5 kilograms, this means there is 1.5 kilograms (1500ml) of excess water in his body. After dialysis, if the patient's weigh drops back to the usual level of 78.5 kilograms, this indicates the patient's body fluid level has reached relative balance. A thorough dialysis can usually make patients feel more comfortable and increase their energy. DRY WEIGHT, which is a patient's original weight, is the weight after eliminating excessive water through dialysis.

20. Why is it necessary we pay attention to hemodialysis patients' blood potassium level?

Potassium has vital functions in maintaining heart, nerve, and muscular functions in the human body. A blood potassium level that is either too high or too low may be dangerous for patients, leading to symptoms of sudden asystole (an irregular heart beat), arrhythmia, (another form of irregular heart beat), muscle weakness and numbness, or muscle cramp. Patients and their families should consult a physician to obtain the patient's blood potassium level in time to make any necessary adjustment in the dietary plan.

21. If the blood potassium level is high, what kind of high potassium foods should the patient avoid?

Please refer to *Appendix One* for "High Potassium Foods."

22 How is it possible to lower the potassium level in vegetables and fruits in cooking?

Potassium dissolves in water easily. When the blood potassium level increases, applying the following methods can reduce the potassium level in vegetables and fruits:

a. Use more water than usual when cooking vegetables, but only eat the vegetable itself, not the resulting liquid.

b. Boil potatoes 2~ 3 times.

c. Boil vegetables before using them in stews, salads, or soup.

d. Avoid using pressure cookers and microwave ovens. (Reheat the food in a wok, repeatedly, instead.)

e. Cut vegetables and fruits into small portions. Eat these frequently, but in small amounts. For instance, cut an apple into 6~8 pieces, and eat 1~2 pieces every 20~30 minutes. Do not eat too much every day.

23. When hyperphosphatemia occurs, what kinds of high phosphorus foods should patients avoid?

High phosphorus foods includes all dairy products, dried beans, whole wheat grains, nuts, peanuts, sesame paste, agar-agar, seaweed, and colas; fruit-favored sodas do not contain high phosphorus. Please refer to *Appendix Two* for "High Phosphorus Foods."

24. How much phosphorus should patients consume daily?

Daily phosphorus intake should be 800~ 1000mg.

25. What are symptoms and signs of hyperphosphatemia?

Pruritus, bone ache, fragilities ossium (fragile small bones), muscle ache, and cardiac function and structural damage are typical of hyperphosphatemia.

26. What is a phosphoric binder?

When blood phosphorous level rise, a doctor will suggest that the patient take a phosphoric binder, such as Tums Renagel or calcium carbonate, to lower blood phosphorus level. After entering the gastrointestinal system, the binder will combine with phosphorus like a sponge, and therefore stops phosphorus from entering the blood stream. It also increases the amount of phosphorus excreted via the stool.

27. Why is it important to eat high quality protein every day?

High quality protein produces less urea when it decomposes in the body compared to other forms of protein. The nitrogenous waste and urea produced by protein decomposition are toxic substances to the human being. But protein is the basis for life, because it maintains the normal functioning of human organs, comprises all kinds of substances vital to the body, repairs human tissues, stimulates growth and development, participates in metabolism, regulates function, and supplies energy. Therefore, after beginning hemodialysis treatment, patients should be aware of daily high quality protein intake. High quality protein is protein that has high biological value, and includes chicken, duck, goose, pork, beef, lamb, fish, milk, and eggs, milk and eggs being the best choices among them. Most cereal protein, as is found in bread and rice, has poorer nutrition value.

28. **When the blood protein level is lower than normal, what kind of food with abundant protein should be eaten? How much should the daily intake be?**

Before beginning dialysis, a patient with a renal problem should eat a low-protein diet, with a protein intake of 0.6 g/kg bodyweight daily. After starting dialysis, protein intake for a hemodialysis patient should be 1.0~1.2g/kg of body weight daily. Protein intake for a peritoneal dialysis patient should be 1.2~1.5g/kg of body weight daily. Please refer to *Appendix Five* for "High Protein Foods."

29. What are dietary differences between hemo-dialysis and peritoneal dialysis patients?

Nutrition	Hemodialysis	Peritoneal dialysis
High-quality protein intake	1.0～1.2 grams/kilogram of body weight daily	1.2～1.5 grams/kilogram of body weight daily
Calories (Kilocalories)	35 kilocalories/ kilogram of body weight daily. For a slim patient without diabetes, this can be raised to 40 kilo-calories/ kilogram of body weight daily.	35 kilocalories/ kilogram of body weight daily. 40 kilocalories/ kilogram of body weight daily for a slim patient with-out diabetes.
Potassium	Should be restrained normally. No limita-tion necessary if blood potassium level is low.	Normally no restraint necessary.
Phosphorus	Need restraint	Need restraint
Sodium	Need restraint	Need restraint
Water	Strictly restrained	Looser restraint than for hemodi-alysis patients

30. What complications do dialysis and peritoneal dialysis patients easily have?

According to a recent U.S. nephrologocial report, hemodialysis and peritoneal dialysis patients can easily have the following complications:

a. Anemia. Patients have symptoms such as weakness, fatigue, and pale complexion.

b. Bone disease. Osteoporosis or osteomalacia.

c. Hypotension or hypertension. Hypotension can occur in hemodialysis patients.

d. Calf muscle or other muscle cramps, muscle aches. These can occur in hemodialysis patients.

e. Febrile reaction. Can occur in hemodialysis patients.

f. Nausea and vomiting. Can occur in hemodialysis patients.

g. Headache, chest, and back pain. Can occur in hemodialysis patients.

h. Pruritus. Can occur in hemodialysis patients

i. Pericarditis. Inflammation of the lining of the heart, caused by inadequate dialysis.

j. Arrhythmia. Can occur in hemodialysis patients.

k. Acidic toxicity. Can be found in association with diabetic end-stage renal disease in patients on dialysis .

l. Hemolysis phenomenon. Can occur in hemo-dialysis patients.

m. Excessive water retention in the body. It can damage the lungs and heart.

n. Hyperkalemia/hypokalemia, hypernatremia/ hyponatremia, hypercalcemia/hypocalcemia, hyperphosphatemia/ hypo- phosphatemia. Can occur in hemodialysis and peritoneal dialysis patients

o. Hypoxemia. Can occur in hemodialysis patients.

p. Neurological system damage. Mostly dam-age to peripheral nerves, and can induce calf muscle ache, discomfort, and numbness.

q. Vascular infection, access infection, perito-neal infection, or arteriovenous shunt infection. Can occur in hemodialysis and peritoneal dialysis patients

r. Anxiety or depression. Can occur in hemodi-alysis and peritoneal dialysis patients.

s. Dementia. Can occur in dialysis patients, aluminum levels high were reported.

t. Protein loss. Can occur in peritoneal dialysis patients.

u. Intracerebral hemorrhage. Can occur in hemodialysis patients.

v. Air embolus. Can occur in hemodialysis patients.

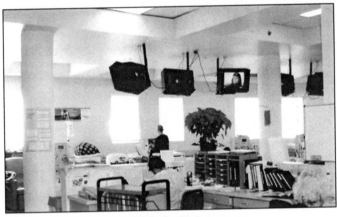

Dialysis Center

31. What are the symptoms when hypercalcemia occurs? What kind of foods should patients avoid?

When hypercalcemia (excessive calcium in the blood) occurs, calcium can leach into soft tissues, causing soft tissue calcification, especially calcification in coronary arteries supplying nutrition to the heart and cardiovalvular tissues, leading to cardiac function damage. Patients have symptoms such as muscle ache and angina. When hypercalcemia occurs, patients should avoid eating high calcium foods. (Please refer to *Appendix Three* for a list of High Calcium Foods)

32. How can osteopathy (bone disease) due to renal failure be prevented by diet?

The kidney excretes an active hormone which can rejuvenate vitamin D needed for bone metabolism. Once renal failure occurs, secretion of this hormone will decrease, causing a drop of vitamin D in the blood. Therefore, bone metabolism cannot function normally and patients may easily suffer complications, such as osteoporosis (bone thinning) and osteomalacia (a bone disease, similar to rickets in children), due to long term hypocalcemia. To prevent these kinds of complications, hemodialysis patients should decrease their daily phosphorus intake and increase their calcium intake. (Please refer to *Appendix Two, "High Phosphorous Foods" and Appendix Three* for High Calcium Foods.) Patients should check if they have a preference for high phosphorus foods, such as dairy items or fish and change their diet to minimize the intake of high phosphorus food and maximize the intake of high calcium food because calcium is an essential mineral for bone formation. According to foreign studies, 70% of long term dialysis patients have complications of malnutrition, including insufficient calcium intake. Besides, phosphorus combines with dietary protein, so patients should check if they are consuming too much protein from food every day.

33. What kind of food should patients eat when anemia occurs?

Renal failure patients tend to have anemia. In addition to injections into the muscle to promote erythropoietin (a chemical that stimulates production of red blood cells) and iron, renal failure patients should consume more high iron, high folic acid, and high vitamin B_{12} foods, such as duck blood, chicken blood, pork liver, turkey liver, razor clams, black sesame, spinach, mushrooms, lichens, and black fungus (high in both iron and potassium).

34. What kinds of vitamins and trace elements do hemodialysis patients tend to lack?

According to studies, hemodialysis patients usually lack vitamin B_1, vitamin B_2, vitamin B_6, vitamin B_{12}, vitamin C, vitamin E, folic acid, biotin, niacin, pantothenic acid, zinc, copper, magnesium, and chromium, due to insufficient food intake, loss of these substances during dialysis, and metabolic abnormality. Patients should pay attention to this problem and take appropriate supplements. Before beginning to take supplements, however, a blood study examination should be carried out to confirm which vitamins or trace elements are deficient, allowing for the correct supplement dosage to be prescribed.

35. What are the dietary principles for diabetic end-stage renal disease patients undergoing hemodialysis?

Patients should establish dietary principles of limiting water and sugar intake, adopting low salt and low fat dietary habits, and consuming high quality protein. (Please refer to above text for how to limit water and salt intake, as well as what high quality protein is and its recommended daily intake. Sugar includes glucose, fructose, and saccharose.

36. What is hemofiltration? What diet and nutrition for hemofiltration patients need?

Hemofiltration is a renal replacement therapy, similar to hemodialysis which is used almost exclusively in the intensive care setting. Thus, almost always used for acute renal failure. It is a slow continuous therapy can be given in outpatient in which sessions usually last 4-5 hours, even longer, and 3 or more times a week. During hemofiltration, a patient's blood is passed through a set of tubing (a filtration circuit) via machine to a semipermeable membrane (the filter) where waste products and water are removed. Replacement fluid is added and the blood is returned to the patient.

The nutrition and diet for hemofiltration patients are the same as hemodialysis patients. To complement what they lack depends on what every patient needs.

37. What is hemodiafiltration?

Hemofiltration is sometimes used in combination with hemodialysis, when it is termed hemodiafiltration. Blood pumped through the blood compartment of a high flux dialyzer, and a high rate of ultrafiltration is used, so there is a high rate of movement of water and solutes from blood to dialysate that must be replaced by substitution fluid that is infused directly into the blood line. However, dialysis solution is also run through the dialysate compartment of the dialyzer. The combination is useful because it results in good removal of both large and small molecular weight solutes.

38. What are the considerations and the precautions during the hemodialysis/hemofiltration?

Considerations:

a. When the patient sleeps, avoid placing pressure on an arm with the access.

b. Do not allow anyone to take a blood pressure reading on an arm with access.

c. Observe the access site after dialysis or hemofiltration, watching for swelling, infection, or bleeding.

d. Do not wear tight clothing around the access site.

e. Routinely check the access site for the "thrill", indicating that the AV site is still functioning. (If the thrill disappears, call your doctor.)

f. Do not use creams or lotions over the access area.

Precautions:

If the patient has an external access, please take additional precautions are as follows,

a. Avoid physical activity that might dislodge the access, which could result in excessive bleeding and air entering the circulatory system. (If it happens, call 911 and get immediate medical attention.)

b. If the blood color in the tube changes and it becomes a dark red, call your health care provider immediately. (The blood may be clotting.)

c. Call you health care provider immediately, if you have a fever or other sign of infection.

APPENDIX ONE

HIGH POTASSIUM FOODS

1. Fruit and its processed products:

Mango, papaya, fresh dates, (except glazed dates and sour dates), peaches, banana, musa, jackfruit, raisins (contain abundant potassium), coconut, dried apricots, dried dates, chestnuts, dried hawthorn, sea buckthorn, dong-ling dates, sweet dates, black dates, dried longan (contains abundant potassium)

2. Seasoning:

Salt substitute with potassium, all kinds of soy sauces (except oyster sauce, which is low in potassium), vinegar (X), mature vinegar, black vinegar, fumigated vinegar (rice vinegar has the lowest potassium level, followed by spiced vinegar and aromatic vinegar), chilli bean sauce, soybean sauce, Pixian chilli sauce, ketchup, thick soy sauce, chili sauce, garlic chilli sauce, spiced salted black beans, sesame paste, spiced cabbage, frissee, ginger, soy-preserved carrot, soy-preserved cucumber, soy-preserved lettuce, dried mustard leaf, carrots, dried turnip, mixed vegetable, soy-preserved garlic, Mongolian leek, flavored ginger, pre-served szechuan pickle, pickled leaf mustard, pickled asparagus (high potassium), pickled salted cabbage, mustard, red chili powder (high in potassium), spiced powder (high in potassium), fennel seed, yeast.

3. Medical foods:

Fresh mint, fresh plantain, fresh divaricate saposhniovia root and its leaf, fresh cassia, fresh perilla leaf, fresh agastachis, fructus lycii, rat snake, cordyceps sinensis。

4. Fat:

Palm seeds.

5. Sweets and glazed fruit:

Chocolate wafer, chocolate, brown sugar (re-fined sugar contains very little potassium.)

6. Beverages:

Tea brick, black tea (high potassium), herbal tea (high potassium), A-graded Long-Jing tea (high po-tassium), green tea (high potassium), guava tea (high potassium), Tieguanyin tea (high potassium), pearl tea, cocoa, malted milk.

7. Instant foods:

Cereals, spiced dried broad beans, potato chips.

8. Snacks and pastries:

Green bean cake, fried chili bean.

9. Baby or infant foods:

Baby milk powder, soybean milk powder, infant milk sponge, infant nutrition powder (infant formula - 5410), simulated breast milk powder.

10. Fish:

Octopus, whelk, conch, dried sea cucumber, salter jelly fish, cuttlefish, dried cuttlefish (high potassium), dried squid (high potassium), dried abalone, dried razor clams, oyster, dried scallops (high potassium), giant tiger prawn, red rail prawns, shrimp, shrimp skin, dried shrimp, crawfish, lizard fish, sole, Spanish mackerelish, halibut, salmon, pomfret, cod, soft-shelled turtle, canned carp, strout, dried sardines, sea robin, spotted sliver scat, big head croaker, topmouth culter, grass carp, carp, tilapia, gymnocypris przewalskii , catfish.

11. Dairy products:

Multiple vitamin milk powder (potassium-rich milk powder), sweetened whole milk powder, whole milk powder, instant whole milk powder, milk tofu, milk granule, butter (food industry), milk tablets.

12. Poultry:

Chicken breast, black-bone chicken, chicken liver, duck gizzard, goose liver, goose gizzard, turkey gizzard, turkey leg, dove.

13. Meat:

Hare, preserved lamb, lamb chops (electric roasted), dried lamb, lean donkey meat, horse meat, beef jerky, curry beef jerky, frozen lamb, lean lamb, frozen goat, sausage, dried meat floss for the elderly, Jinhua ham, beef brain, Taicang dried meat floss, Cantonese sausage, barbecued pork, preserved meat, salted meat, dried pork floss, pork fillet, lean pork, pork liver, pork gallbladder.

14. Nuts and seeds:

Jackfruit seed, walnuts, pecans, chesnuts, fried pine nuts, pine nuts, almonds, cashews, fried hazelnuts, sesame, peanuts (roasted or raw), dried hazelnuts (high potassium), sunflower seeds (roasted or raw), dried lotus seeds, fried pumpkin seeds, fried watermelon seeds, watermelon seeds with plum flavor, black sesame powder.

15. Fungus:

Dried black mushroom (high potassium), dried golden oyster mushroom (high potassium), mongolia mushroom (white sanctity mushroom, high potassium), dried mushroom (high potassium), straw mushroom, black fungus, mushroom, dried chinese mushroom, morel (high potassium), white fungus (high potassium), pseudo honey mushroom (high potassium), water-soaked honey mushroom, dried seaweed, dried algae, dried agar-agar (high potassium).

16. Vegetables:

Persimmon, carrot, dehydrated carrot (high potassium), fava beans, peas (with pod), green soy bean, chili pepper (high potassium), dehydrated bell pepper (high potassium), dried marrow, pumpkin powder, serpent gourd, garlic, purple skin garlic, dehydrated garlic, red skin onion, dehydrated pink skin onion, dehydrated onion, dehydrated cabbage, dehydrated rape, dehydrated broccoli, mustard leaf, spinach, spinach (without root), baby carrot, baby turnip, beet leaf, dehydrated caraway (high potassium), red edible amaranth, bamboo shoot, dried bamboo shoot (high potassium), summer and fall bamboo shot, spring bamboo shoot, bamboo shoot, lily (fresh and dried), dehydrated lily, endive, arrowhead, water caltrop, water chestnut, taro, flavored ginger, mugwort, sweet potato leaf, thyme, yellow patrinia herb, heartleaf houttuynia (high potassium), belvedere, bamboo, garden cress, jute leaf, basil, oregano, salsify, dandelion leaf, fennel corm, edible rhubarb, edible jute, lemon grass , heartleaf houttuynia, clethra loosestrife herb, zie-xiangcha vege, alfalfa.

17. Potato, starches and their products:

Potato, potato powder (high potassium), dried sweet potato, cassava, Taro powder.

18. Dried bean curd products:

Soybean (high potassium), black bean (high potassium), soybean powder (high potassium), fermented soy bean (high potassium), bean pulp (high potassium), bean curd sheet, dried bean curd sticks, dried bean curd, green beans, green bean noodles (high potassium), adzuki beans, red kidney beans, purple beans, red kidney beans (high potassium), kidney beans with skin (high potassium), fava beans (high potassium), fava beans with skin, skinless fava beans, roasted fava beans (high potassium), big beans (brain bean), fried fava beans, hyacinth beans (high potassium), black-eyed beans, cow peas, purple cow peas, peas.

19. Cereals:

Wheat germ, whole wheat, corn noodle, highland barley, bitter soba powder, soba, corn wheat noodle.

Appendix Two

High Phosphorus Foods

1. Cereals:
Wheat germ powder, whole wheat, black rice, brown rice, soba, highland barley.

2. Potato, starches, and their products:
Taro powder

3. Dried bean curd products:
Soybeans, black beans, peas, soybean powder, tofu stripe, bean curd roll, tofu skin, fried bean curd puff, dried bean curd sticks, bean curd stick, thin sheets of bean curd, mung bean noodles, adzuki beans, kidney beans, fava beans with skin, maya potatoes, big beans (brain bean), roasted fava beans, fried fava beans, white hyacinth beans, black-eyed beans, cow peas, purple cow peas, gorse beans, red incienso, mung beans.

4. Vegetables:
Fresh fava beans, green soy beans, hot peppers, pumpkin powder, dehydrated garlic, dehydrated cabbage, dehydrated spinch, dried bamboo shoot, dried

black bamboo, lily bud, artemisia aphaerocephala krasch seed, agriophyllum pungens, alfalfa seed.

5. Fungus:

Russula rubra, dried black mushrooms, dried mushrooms, dried agaric (black fungus), dried Chinese mushrooms, tremella, algae, agar-agar, morel (high phosphorus), mongolia mushrooms (white sanctity mushroom, high phosphorus).

6. Fruit:

Hawthorn, dried black berries, dried longan.

7. Nuts and seeds:

Dried walnuts, dried Chinese walnuts, cooked Chinese walnuts, raw pine seeds, fried pine seeds, pine seeds, dried almonds, whole almonds, cashews, dried filberts, roasted filberts, sesame, peanuts, sunflower seeds, dried lotus seeds, watermelon seeds, white sesame, black sesame, pumpkin seeds (high phosphorus.)

8. Meat:

Beef brain, beef jerky, sheep liver, sheep brain, dried lamb, horse meet, hare.

9. Poultry:

Sand grouse, chicken liver, fried chicken, duck gizzard, canned stewed duck, turkey leg.

10. Dairy products:

Whole milk powder, milk tofu, milk granule, Chedder cheese, goat cheese, milk skin, milk tablets, whole milk powder, cheese, sweetened whole milk powder (high phosphorus), Tibetan cheese (high phosphorus)

11. Egg products:

Yolk, custard powder, yolk powder, preserved egg, salted duck eggs, quail eggs.

12. Fish:

Topmouth culter, grass carp, carp, loach, banded reef cod (grouper), Gymnocypris przewalskii , canned carp, river eel, sea robin, Mandarin fish, bass, matreel, caviar, estuarine tapertail anchovy, halibut, grass carp, trout, dried fish fillet, ornate spiny lobster, giant tiger prawn, red rail prawn, Chinese prawn, prawn, shrimp, lobster, grass shrimp, tiger shrimp, shelled dried shrimp, red claw, abalone (dried), dried razor clams, dried cuttlefish, dried squid, wrasses, dried sardines, lizard fish, cray fish, river mussels, salted tench, cod.

13. Snacks and Pastries:
Pancake, fried noodle with highland barley, fried broad beans, corn crisps

14. Instant foods:
Oatmeal, cereal, calcium milk cookies, calcium cookies.

15. Beverages:
Black tea, herbal tea, A-graded Long-Jing tea, Tieguanyin tea, pearl tea, ice cream powder, cocoa.

16. Fats:
Palm oil.

17. Seasonings:
Flavored soy sauce, refined soy sauce, thick soy sauce, sesame paste, fermented spicy bean curd, fermented bean curd, mustard, red chili pepper powder, fennel seed, sweet vinegar, black vinegar, fumigated vinegar, soy sauce, yeast, wild pepper, dried yeast (high phosphorus.)

18. Medical food:

Grosvenor momordica fruit, grand Torreya seeds, fresh plantain seeds, fructus lycii, frog, silkworm chrysalis, scorpion, agastachis.

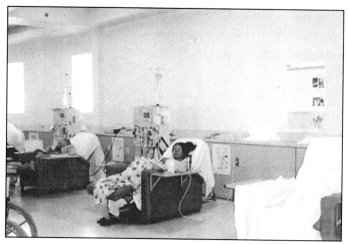

Dialysis Center

Appendix Three

High Calcium Foods

1. Beans and bean products:

Black beans, soybeans, peas, soybean powder, bean curd strips, thin sheets of bean curd, dried bean curd, fermented tofu, soy-sauce-flavored dried bean curd, stewed dried tofu, bean curd, dried bean curd (high calcium), vegetarian large gut, vegetarian chicken, deep fried vegetarian shrimp, purple beans, kidney beans (with skin), brain beans, fava beans, roasted fava beans, blossom out beans, gorse beans, red incienso.

2. Vegetables:

Dehydrated carrot, pink skin onion (dehydrated), dehydrated cabbage, dehydrated spinch, baby carrot, baby turnip, dehydrated caraway, shepherd's purse, lily bud, artemisia aphaerocephala krasch seed, yellow patrinia herb, thyme, cephalanoplos segetum, pea sprout, pea, hound's tongue, vicia sativa, belvedere, bamboo, juteleaf, salsola colfina (suaeda glauca bunge), basil (common bluebeard), oregano, bordock leaf, stone veges, dandelion leaf, cudweed herb, adenophora hunanensis leaf, edible ephedra, aizoon stonecrop herb, vicia unijuga, sweet morning glory, common dayflower herb, wild leek, artemisia capillaris thunb, field sowthistle herb, alfalfa, alfalfa seeds, braken fern (dehydrated), wild amaranth, zie xiangcha veges.

3. Fungus:
Agaric, morel, black moss, seaweed, dried agar-agar

4. Fruits:
Spine dates, blackberries (dried)

5. Nuts:
Almonds, roasted filberts, sesame, roasted peanuts, white sesame, black sesame

6. Dairy products:
Instant milk, sweetened whole milk powder, whole milk powder, cheese, milk tofu, milk granule (dried cheese), Tibetan cheese, yorgot , goat cheese, butter residue , butter , condensed milk, milk skin, milk tablets, Cheddar cheese (whole or fat free).

7. **Eggs and egg products:**
Custard powder, yolk powder.

8. **Fish:**
Loach, canned carp, shelled dried shrimp, shrimp, grass shrimp, shrimp skin, shelled dried shrimp, prawn brain, sea crab, serrated mud crab, swimming crab, crab meat, abalone, river mussel, whelk, periwinkle, river snail (high calcium), winkle (high calcium), sea cucumber, dried sardines.

9. **Snacks and Pastries:**
Uncongealed tofu, corn crisps, Liao-Hua drop, calcium cookies.

10. **Beverages:**
Tea brick, black tea, herbal tea, A-graded Long-Jing tea, green tea, Tieguanyin tea, pearl tea, ice cream powder, guava tea (high calcium)

11. **Sweets and glazed fruits:**
Preserved apricots, watermelon skin candy.

12. **Fats:**
Palm seed powder.

13. Seasonings:

Soy sauce (monosodium gultamate), spicy broad bean sauce, sesame paste (high calcium), Guilin preserved bean curd , dried Guilin turnip, dried mustard leaf (high calcium), Mongolian leek, pickled cabbage, wild pepper, Huang-Mao seed, mustard, sophora alopecuroides, fennel seed, lake salt.

14. Medical foods:

Mint, fresh schisandra leaf, fresh plantain seeds and fresh plantain, licorice root, safflower, chrysanthemum morifolium, fresh cassia, fresh perilla leaf, agastachis and fresh agastachis (including leaf).

APPENDIX FOUR

HIGH SODIUM FOODS

1. Cereals:
Dried noodles, shrimp-flavored noodles, cruller, and twisted cruller.

2. Dried bean curd products:
Fried bean curd strips, dried bean curd, vegetarian ham, vegetarian chicken, vegetarian's delight, deep fried vegetarian shrimp (high sodium), deep fried fava beans (blossom out beans).

3. Vegetables:
Dehydrated carrot, tomato (fresh or canned), dehydrated spinch, Swiss chard, dehydrated caraway (high sodium).

4. Fungus:
Canned lily bud, dried seaweed, agar, dried algae (algae strips, high sodium, 4955mg sodium per 100g), dried agar-agar.

5. Fruit:

Flattened preserved mandarin orange.

6. Nuts and seeds:

Dried Chinese walnuts , cooked walnuts, dried almonds (roasted with salt), roasted peanuts, roasted sunflower seeds (high sodium, 1322mg sodium per 100g).

7. Meat:

Pork liver, pork gallbladder, barbecued pork, canned fried diced chicken, bacon, spiced pork haslet, Spam® luncheon meat, canned fillet stripes, stewed pork liver, cooked pork hoof, boiled pork elbow, dried pork floss, Fujianese dried meat floss (high sodium), dried meat floss for the elderly (high sodium, 2301mg sodium per 100g), Taicang dried meat floss (high sodium), tea-flavored gut, preserved sausage (high sodium), gut (high sodium), gut flavored with egg albumen (high sodium), dried gut, Cantonese sausage (high sodium), hawthorn gut, ham, preserved gut (high sodium), Songjingese gut, garlic-flavored gut, sausage (high sodium, 2309mg sodium per 100g), canned sausage, hot dogs, small paste ham, canned gut, canned tripes (294mg sodium per 100g), square ham, ham (high sodium), Jinhua ham (233mg sodium per 100g), round ham, beef-flavored sauce, canned braised beef, beef jerky (412mg sodium per 100g), curry beef jerky (high sodium, 2075 233mg sodium per 100g), dried beef floss (high sodium), lamb blood, preserved lamb (high sodium, 8991mg sodium per 100g), cooked lamb, electric roasted lamb, roasted lamb, deep-fried lamb, goat-flavored sauce, stewed donkey meat.

8. Poultry:

Grilled chicken (1000mg sodium per 100g), roasted chicken, fried chicken, canned braised duck, canned sauced duck, cooked salted duck (high sodium, 1557mg sodium per 100g).

9. Dairy products:

Multiple vitamin milk powder, sweetened whole milk powder, cheese (dried cheese), Cheddar cheese (including regular and fat free), whole-fat soft cheese, goat cheese (high sodium, 1440mg sodium per 100g).

10. Egg products:

Egg powder, preserved eggs, salted duck eggs (high sodium, 2706mg sodium per 100g), canned quail eggs.

11. Fish:

Canned carp (high sodium, 2310mg sodium per 100g), dried sardines (high sodium, 4375mg sodium per 100g), caviar (high sodium), dried fish fillet (high sodium, 2300mg sodium per 100g), Thai fish sauce (high sodium), prawn, shelled dried shrimp (high sodium, 5057mg sodium per 100g), dried small shrimps (high sodium, 4891mg sodium per 100g), shrimp brain sauce, swimming crab, dried abalone (high sodium), dried razor clams (high sodium), oyster shell , oysters, granular ark, scallops, dried scallops, silvery short-neck clams, mussels, clams (X), short-neck clams, ark shell, autumn clams, sea cucumber, dried sea cucumber, salted jellyfish, dried cuttlefish, dried squid.

12. Snacks and pastries:

Bai shui yangtou, spring roll, Jiao quan, fried lobster chips, glazed bread twist, niang pi, deep fried broad beans, banyou su bing, fried chicken leg, puff.

13. Instant Foods:

Instant noodles (high sodium, 1144 mg sodium per 100g), multiple vitamins bread, croissants, wheat bread, milk cookies, soda cookies, wafers.

14. Beverages:

Vegetable juice.

15. Seasonings:

All kinds of soy sauces (high sodium, 2000-6000mg sodium per 100g), mature vinegar, black vinegar, fumigated vinegar, spiced salted black bean, *broad bean sauce, *spicy broad bean sauce, *peanut paste, *soybean sauce, *thick soy sauce, *tabasco, *hot chili sauce, *beef-flavored spicy sauce, *garlic chili sauce, *sweet sauce, *spiced chili sauce, *Pixian chilli sauce, preserved bean curd, fermented preserved bean curd (fermented tofu), fermented spicy bean curd, Guilin preserved bean curd, seasoned preserved bean curd (various preserved bean curd contains rich sodium, too)
(* rich sodium)

All kinds of pickled vegetables and salted vegetables (contain rich sodium).

Rice powder for steamed meat also contains rich sodium.

All kinds of salt, including lake salt, fine salt, and earth salt, contain rich sodium. For example, every 100g lake salt contains 92768mg sodium.

Monosodium gultamate (contain high sodium, 8160mg sodium per 100g)

Appendix Five

High Protein Foods

Protein (g)/per 100g

Beef (fillet)	22.2	Roasted chicken	22.4	Shark	22.2
Beef (fore-tendon)	20.3	Fried chicken	20.3	Pomfret	18.5
Beef hoof thew(?)	34.1	Duck web	26.9	Snapper	17.9
Pork (fillet)	20.2	Quail	20.2	Small estuarine taper tail anchovy	15.5
Lean pork	20.3	Mackerel	20.1	Turbot (flounder)	21.1
Pork leg	17.9	Hairtail	17.7	Cod	20.4
Pork hoof thew	35.3	Crucian carp	17.1	Kuai fish (Lifish)	20.7
Curry beef jerky	45.9	Silver carp	17.8	Legen-dary turtle	20.2
Lamb neck	21.3	Catfish	17.3	Chinese prawn	18.3
Lamb fillet	20.5	Gymnoc ypris przewals	17.8	Yellow eel	18.0

		kii			
Lamb (blue sheep)	21.3	Grouper	18.5	Soft-shelled turtle	17.8
Lamb hoof thew(?) (not dried)	8.4	Bream	18.3	Frog	20.5
Lamb (cooked)	23.2	Mandarin fish	19.9	Snake	15.1
Lamb chops (electric roasted)	26.4	Trout	18.6	Prawn	18.6
Lamb chops (roasted)	36	Silver Carp Fish	15.3	Sea prawn	16.8
Boiled mutton	27.3	Wrasses	17.6	Shrimp	16.4
Goat (sauce)	25.4	Carp	18.4	Greasy-back shrimp	18.2
Donkey meat (sauce)	33.7	Sea eel	18.8	River shrimp	10.3
Donkey meat (stewed)	27.7	Large yellow Croaker	17.9	Lobster	18.9
Donkey meat (cooked)	27	Yellow croaker	17.9	Red claw	14.8
Horse meat (stewed)	30.5	Leather jacket	18.1	Sea crab	13.8
Camel hoof	25.6	Big head croaker	18.9	River crab	17.5

Camel hoof	72.8	Mackerel	21.2	Swimming crab	15.9
Wild chicken	20.8	Brown barracuda	15.9	Razor clams	7.3
Sandgrouse	20.0	Flounder	20.8	Ark shell	13.9
Chicken claw	23.9	Bass	18.6	Mud mussel	10.9
Grill chicken	29.6	Matreel	19.9	Oyster	10.9
Scallops	11.1	Mung beans	21.6	Sprouted beans	12.4
Silvery short- neck clams	12.2	Adzuki beans	20.2	Dried black bamboo shot	17.6
Field whelk	19.8	Runner beans (red)	19.1	Dried black fungus	12.1
Snail	7.5	Kidney beans (white)	23.4	Dried Chinese mushroom	20.0
Mud snails	11.0	Soy beans	35.0	Chinese mushroom	2.2
Conch (win-kle)	22.7	Black peas	36.0	Tremella	10.0
Squid	17.0	Cow peas	19.3	Dried black moss	20.2

Deep fried broad beans	25.1	Peas	20.3	Dried agar-agar	26.7
Oatmeal	15.0	Green soy bean	13.1	Chesnut	4.2
Black tea	26.7	Soy beans	32.7	Soba	9.3
Herbal tea	27.1	Soybean powder	19.7	Coix seed	12.8
Persimmon leaf tea	25.8	Bean pulp	42.5	Roasted wheat	20.4
Pearl tea	28.7	Tofu (northern Chinese style)	12.2	Ginkgo seed	13.2
Cacoa	20.9	Tofu (southern Chinese style)	6.2	Pecans	12.8
Sesame paste	19.2	Soy milk	2.4	Walnuts	14.8
Sugared instant whole milk	22.5	Soybean milk	1.8	Rough walnuts	12.0
Yogurt	2.5	Bean curd stripes	21.5	Pine seeds (raw)	12.6
Milk	3.0	Bean curd sheet	44.6	Pine kernels	13.4

Tibetan cheese	39.1	Fried bean curd puff	17.0	Almonds	22.5
Broad bean sauce	13.6	Dried bean curd sticks	44.6	Peanuts	12.0
Black sesame	19.1	Thin sheets of bean curd	24.5	Dried filberts	20.0
Soybean sauce	12.1	Dried bean curd (X)	16.2	Peanuts	24.8
Mustard	23.6	Bean curd	15.8	Fried peanuts	23.9
Fava beans with skin	24.6	Fried gluten puff	26.9	Fried sunflower seeds	22.6
Maya beans	25.4	Gluten	23.5	Sunflower seeds	19.1
Bain beans	23.4	Smoked bean curd	15.8	Dried lotus seeds	17.2
Hyacinth beans	25.3	Vegetarian chicken	16.5	Pumpkin seeds	33.2
White hyacinth beans	19.0	Vegetar-ian's delight	14.0	Watermelon seeds	33.4

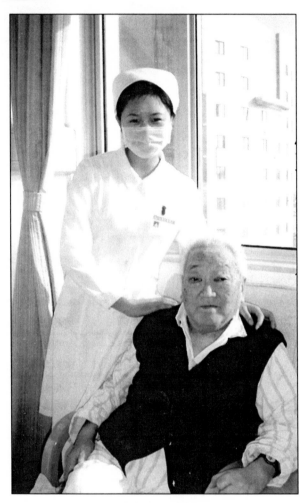

Dialysis Patient

BIOGRAPHY

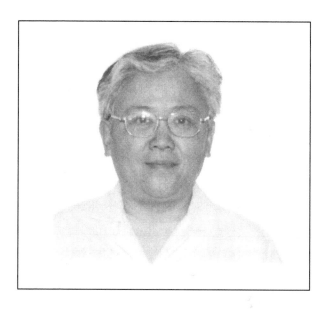

Shuang Chen, M.D., R.H.(AHG) is an experienced practitioner in Chinese & Western herbal medicine combined with homeopathic medicine in the US. She is also an experienced dermatologist & mycologist in China and Japan. Dr. Chen graduated from the Fourth Military Medical University in China 34 years ago, and had further study in Teikyo University, Medical School, Dept. of Dermatology & Mycology in Japan in the 80's. She is a member of The Japanese Society for Investigative Dermatology.

Dr. Chen has devoted her practice to natural medicine, and has favored herbal medicine and nutrition over the past 15 years. Dr. Chen focuses on the search for effective therapies using Oriental & Western herbal medicine and nutrition to treat skin diseases, venereal diseases and fungal infected disorders. She had distant study in homeopathic medicine and obtained a Master Herbalist Diploma from the Australasian College of Healthy Sciences in Portland, Oregon of the US.

Dr. Chen is a Registered Herbalist in the US. Besides being a member of the American Botanical Council, a member of the American Herbalist Guild and a member of the Delta Epsilon Tau in the US, she is also a medical research writer.

Donglian Cai, M.D., Ph.D. is a nationally renowned professor in nutriology in China.

Dr. Donglian Cai is Chairman of the Department of Clinical Nutriology, Changhai Hospital, which is a teaching hospital of The Second Military Medical University, Shanghai, China; he is Vice Chairman of the Clinical Nutriology Brach of the Shanghai Nutrition Society(SNS); Vice Chairman of the Nutrition and Food therapy Brach of the China Association of Chinese Medicine(CACM);

and Standing Director of the Parenteral & Enteral Nutrition Branch of the Chinese Medical Association(CAM).

Dr. Donglian Cai wrote a series of books in nutriology in China, and his APPLIED NUTRIOLOGY which is a highly authoritative professional book in medical field and an important reference book for clinical nutriologists and other professionals, which was published in Hong Kong and China.